Tantric Massage for Beginners

Awaken Your Senses, Deepen Intimacy, and Discover the Art of Sensual Connection

Lewis Finan

Table of Contents

Introduction

In the intricate tapestry of human connection, the realm of sensuality and intimacy holds a profound significance. As we navigate the complexities of modern life, it becomes increasingly important to explore avenues that allow us to deepen our connections with ourselves and our partners. Within this exploration lies the ancient and sacred art of tantric massage—a practice that transcends the physical, delving into the realms of spiritual and emotional connection.

Welcome to "Tantric Massage for Beginners: Awaken Your Senses, Deepen Intimacy, and Discover the Art of Sensual Connection." This book is a gentle yet empowering guide designed for those who seek to embark on a transformative journey into the world of tantric massage. Whether you are an individual looking to enhance your connection with your own body or a couple seeking to reignite the flame of passion, this book offers a comprehensive introduction to the principles and techniques that form the foundation of tantric massage.

As we delve into the pages of this guide, we will unravel the mystique surrounding tantric practices, demystifying misconceptions and providing practical insights into the art of sensual connection. Drawing inspiration from ancient Eastern traditions and combining them with contemporary understanding, this book serves as a bridge between the timeless wisdom of tantra and the demands of our modern lives.

In the chapters that follow, we will explore the fundamental principles of tantric massage, from creating the right environment and establishing trust to the intricacies of touch and breath. Each concept is presented in a manner that caters to beginners, allowing for a gradual and enjoyable progression into the world of tantric exploration.

Embrace the opportunity to reawaken your senses, fostering a deeper connection with yourself and your partner. Discover the transformative power of tantric massage as a pathway to increased intimacy, heightened awareness, and a more profound understanding of the intricate dance between body, mind, and spirit.

Let this book be your guide as you embark on a journey that goes beyond the physical, inviting you to explore the vast landscape of sensuality and connection. May it inspire you to embrace the beauty of the present moment, fostering a more profound and authentic connection with yourself and your beloved.

Are you ready to embark on this sensual odyssey? The adventure begins now.

Understanding Tantra

At its core, Tantra is far more than a set of ancient techniques; it is a philosophy that embraces the holistic integration of mind, body, and spirit. Originating from ancient Eastern traditions, particularly in Hinduism and Buddhism, Tantra is a path that seeks to transcend the ordinary and connect with the divine essence within and around us.

Contrary to common misconceptions, Tantra extends beyond the realm of sexuality. It encompasses a wide array of practices aimed at expanding consciousness, deepening self-awareness, and fostering a profound connection with the universe. Tantra encourages individuals to embrace life in its entirety, recognizing the sacredness inherent in every aspect of existence.

One of the key tenets of Tantra is the idea that everything is interconnected and divine. Rather than viewing the world in terms of dualities, such as good and bad or sacred and profane, Tantra encourages us to see the unity that underlies all apparent opposites. This perspective is foundational to understanding the transformative potential of Tantra.

In the context of intimacy and sensuality, Tantra introduces a unique approach that goes beyond the mere physical act. It invites us to cultivate a mindful presence, elevating the act of love-making to a sacred and spiritual experience. Within the realm of Tantra, sexual energy is considered a potent force that, when harnessed consciously, can lead to profound states of ecstasy, spiritual awakening, and deep connection.

Tantric practices often involve rituals, meditations, and specific breathwork techniques to channel and amplify the flow of energy within the body. These practices aim to awaken dormant potentials, break down barriers, and facilitate a harmonious flow of energy throughout the entire being.

It is crucial to recognize that Tantra is a highly individual and experiential path. What works for one person may not resonate with another. Therefore, Tantra invites exploration and adaptation, encouraging practitioners to discover their unique path within the broader framework of its principles.

In the chapters that follow, we will delve into the world of Tantric massage, a practice that embodies the essence of Tantra's holistic approach to intimacy. As we explore the principles and techniques of Tantric massage, remember that this is just one facet of a vast and rich tradition. Approach this journey with an open heart and a willingness to embrace the transformative potential that Tantra offers.

The Essence of Tantric Massage

Tantric massage is a profound and ancient practice that transcends the boundaries of conventional touch, inviting individuals and couples to explore the depths of intimacy, sensuality, and spiritual connection. Rooted in the principles of Tantra, this artful form of massage is a gateway to unlocking the hidden dimensions of pleasure, self-discovery, and profound connection.

At its essence, Tantric massage is more than a skillful manipulation of the body; it is an intentional and sacred dance between giver and receiver, a journey into the realms of heightened awareness and conscious touch. Unlike conventional massages that primarily focus on physical tension relief, Tantric massage aims to awaken the dormant energies within, fostering a harmonious balance of body, mind, and spirit.

Conscious Presence:

A cornerstone of Tantric massage is the cultivation of conscious presence. Both the giver and receiver are encouraged to be fully present at the moment, shedding distractions and preconceptions. This heightened awareness creates a sacred space where the exchange of energy becomes a deeply spiritual communion.

Breathwork and Energy Flow:

Tantric massage incorporates deliberate breathwork to synchronize the rhythm of breath between the participants. This synchronization serves as a gateway to accessing and directing the flow of vital life energy, known as "prana" or "chi." Through intentional breath, practitioners amplify and circulate this energy, creating a profound connection that extends beyond the physical realm.

Honoring the Body as a Temple:

In Tantric philosophy, the body is revered as a sacred vessel, a temple that houses the divine. Tantric massage approaches the body with deep reverence, recognizing every inch as a landscape deserving of attention, adoration, and respect. The massage becomes a celebration of the body's beauty, inviting a sense of profound self-love and acceptance.

Transcending Boundaries:

Tantric massage challenges societal taboos surrounding touch and intimacy. It encourages participants to release inhibitions and surrender to the experience, creating an atmosphere of trust and vulnerability. Within this sacred space, individuals can explore the edges of their comfort zones, transcending self-imposed limitations.

Healing and Transformation:

Beyond the realm of pleasure, Tantric massage is recognized for its potential to facilitate healing and transformation. By consciously engaging with the body's energy centers, known as chakras, and by releasing stored emotional and energetic blockages, practitioners often experience a profound sense of release, renewal, and rejuvenation.

In the chapters that follow, we will embark on a journey into the heart of Tantric massage, exploring techniques, rituals, and the art of conscious touch. Whether you are a beginner seeking to deepen your connection with self and others or a seasoned explorer of Tantra, may this exploration guide you toward a richer, more fulfilling experience of intimacy and sensuality? The essence of Tantric massage lies not only in its techniques but in the mindful and heartful connection it fosters—a connection that has the potential to awaken the divine within and around us.

Chapter 1: Preparing for the Journey

Before embarking on the transformative journey of Tantric massage, it is essential to lay the foundation for a sacred and intentional space. Preparation is key, as it sets the stage for a profound exploration of sensuality and connection. In this chapter, we will delve into the necessary steps to ensure a harmonious and mindful beginning to your Tantric massage experience.

1. Creating the Sacred Space:

The environment in which Tantric massage takes place plays a crucial role in setting the tone for the experience. Designate a space that is clean, comfortable, and free from distractions. Consider using soft lighting, candles, and soothing music to create an ambiance that fosters relaxation and mindfulness.

2. Establishing Trust and Communication:

Trust is the cornerstone of any Tantric experience. Whether you are the giver or receiver, take the time to establish clear communication and mutual trust with your partner. This includes discussing boundaries, desires, and any concerns that may arise during the massage. Open dialogue ensures a safe and consensual exploration.

3. Cultivating Mindful Presence:

Begin by centering yourself through mindful breathing and presence. As the giver, take a moment to connect with your intentions and energy. As the receiver, focus on grounding yourself in the present moment, releasing any expectations, and surrendering to the experience. This shared mindfulness creates a powerful energetic connection between participants.

4. Connecting with Breath:

Conscious breathwork is a fundamental aspect of Tantric massage. Encourage synchronized breathing between the giver and receiver to establish a harmonious energetic flow. Deep, intentional breaths not only enhance relaxation but also serve as a bridge to deeper states of connection and intimacy.

5. Honoring Consent and Boundaries:

Respect for boundaries is paramount in Tantric massage. Prioritize open communication and continuously check in with your partner throughout the experience. Establish a system of verbal or non-verbal cues to ensure that both participants feel safe and comfortable at all times.

6. Rituals of Purification:

Consider incorporating rituals of purification before the massage begins. This may involve a shared shower or a ceremonial cleansing to symbolize the shedding of inhibitions and the preparation for a sacred exchange of energy.

7. Setting Intentions:

Before the journey unfolds, take a moment to set intentions for the experience. Consider what you wish to explore, discover, or release. Shared intentions can align the energies of both participants, creating a purposeful and transformative space.

As you prepare for the Tantric massage journey, remember that the essence of this practice lies in conscious awareness, trust, and the celebration of the sacredness of the body. In the upcoming chapters, we will delve into the practical aspects of Tantric massage techniques, guiding you through a step-by-step exploration of this ancient art form. May your preparations lay the groundwork for a profound and enriching experience of sensuality and connection.

1.1 Creating the Right Atmosphere

The atmosphere in which Tantric massage unfolds is not merely a backdrop; it is a vital element that shapes the energy and intention of the experience. In this chapter, we will explore the art of creating the right atmosphere—a sacred space that invites participants into a journey of heightened senses, connection, and self-discovery.

1. Sacred Space Design:

Crafting a sacred space is the first step toward a transformative Tantric massage experience. Choose a room that is private, quiet, and free from external disruptions. Consider using soft, indirect lighting such as candles or dim lamps to create a warm and intimate ambiance. The goal is to evoke a sense of tranquility and openness.

2. Sensory Elements:

Engage the senses to deepen the overall experience. Experiment with aromatherapy by using essential oils such as lavender or sandalwood to promote relaxation. Select soothing music with a gentle rhythm to enhance the auditory atmosphere. Soft fabrics and cushions can contribute to the tactile comfort of the space.

3. Temperature and Comfort:

Maintain a comfortable temperature in the room, as warmth fosters relaxation. Ensure that the massage surface, whether a bed or a massage table, is draped with soft, clean linens. Attend to details such as cushions and blankets to provide optimal comfort for both the giver and receiver.

4. Energetic Clearing:

Before the massage begins, consider engaging in a brief ritual to energetically clear the space. This may involve burning sage or palo santo, visualizing a purifying light, or simply setting an intention for the space to be filled with positive and loving energy.

5. Connection with Nature:

If possible, incorporate elements of nature into the space. Fresh flowers, potted plants, or natural crystals can infuse the environment with grounding and revitalizing energy. Nature has a way of harmonizing and enhancing the energetic flow of the space.

6. Limiting Distractions:

Turn off electronic devices, and minimize external distractions to create a sanctuary free from interruptions. The intention is to foster a deep sense of presence, allowing both the giver and receiver to fully immerse themselves in the unfolding experience.

7. Sacred Symbols and Artifacts:

Consider adding sacred symbols or meaningful artifacts to the space. This could be a representation of a deity, a personal totem, or symbols that hold significance for both participants. These elements can serve as focal points for intention-setting and energetic connection.

8. Mutual Preparation:

Both the giver and receiver should participate in preparing the space. This collaborative effort not only enhances the shared experience but also deepens the connection between participants. As you collectively engage in setting the stage, you lay the groundwork for a harmonious and resonant atmosphere.

Creating the right atmosphere is an art in itself, a dance between the tangible and the subtle. As you infuse intention into the space, you pave the way for a Tantric massage experience that transcends the physical, reaching into the realms of the spiritual and the profound. In the next chapter, we will delve into the practical aspects of initiating touch and exploring the intricate dance of energy that Tantric massage unfolds.

1.3 Setting Intentions

Intentions act as the compass guiding the journey of Tantric massage, infusing the experience with purpose and direction. In this chapter, we explore the significance of setting intentions before diving into the intricacies of touch and connection. By clarifying your individual and shared intentions, you cultivate a transformative space for self-discovery, healing, and deep connection.

1. Personal Reflection:

Begin by individually reflecting on your intentions for the Tantric massage experience. What aspects of yourself or your relationship do you wish to explore or enhance? Consider personal desires, emotional needs, or areas of self-discovery. Allow these reflections to be the seeds from which your intentions will grow.

2. Shared Intentions:

Once each participant has clarified their intentions, come together to discuss and formulate shared intentions for the Tantric massage session. This collaborative process creates a unified energy and aligns both individuals with a common purpose. Shared intentions foster a sense of connection and mutual understanding.

3. Clarity and Specificity:

Craft intentions that are clear, specific, and positive. Instead of vague aspirations, articulate your desires with precision. For example, rather than stating a general intention like "to relax," you might express the intention as "to cultivate a deep sense of relaxation that permeates both body and mind."

4. Affirmative Language:

Frame your intentions in affirmative language. Use words that express what you want to invite into the experience rather than what you wish to avoid. Positive affirmations set the tone for a constructive and empowering exploration.

5. Emotional and Spiritual Aspects:

Consider intentions that delve into the emotional and spiritual realms. Tantric massage is not solely a physical experience; it is an opportunity for emotional release, spiritual connection, and self-discovery. Explore intentions related to opening the heart, deepening trust, or connecting on a soul level.

6. Flexibility and Surrender:

While setting intentions is essential, remain open to the fluidity of the experience. Allow space for spontaneity, organic connection, and the possibility of unexpected insights. Intentions serve as a guide, but the beauty of Tantric massage often lies in the moments of unscripted connection.

7. Ritual of Setting Intentions:

Consider incorporating a brief ritual for setting intentions before the massage begins. This could involve a shared meditation, spoken affirmations, or a simple exchange of words expressing your hopes and desires for the session. Rituals enhance the sacredness of the space and deepen the energetic connection.

8. Revisiting Intentions:

Throughout the Tantric massage experience, revisit your intentions as a way to realign and refocus your energy. This can be done silently through internal reflection or shared verbally between the giver and receiver. Acknowledge the unfolding journey and celebrate the moments that resonate with your intentions.

Setting intentions infuses your Tantric massage with purpose and mindfulness, transforming it from a physical exchange into a profound exploration of self and connection. As you move forward into the subsequent chapters, keep these intentions as beacons, guiding you through the dance of touch, breath, and energetic exchange.

Chapter 2: The Fundamentals of Tantric Massage

With the foundation laid and intentions set, we now delve into the heart of Tantric massage—the fundamental principles and techniques that distinguish it as a sacred and transformative practice. In this chapter, we explore the intricate dance of touch, breath, and energetic connection that defines the art of Tantric massage.

1. Mindful Touch:

Tantric massage is more than a sequence of physical movements; it is a dance of mindful touch. The giver approaches the receiver's body with reverence, awareness, and intention. Each stroke, caress, or press is a communication that transcends words, fostering a deep connection between the giver and receiver.

2. Conscious Breathwork:

Integrate conscious breathwork into the massage experience. Encourage synchronized breathing between the giver and receiver to harmonize energies and deepen the connection. Breath serves as a bridge between the physical and the spiritual, amplifying the flow of vital life energy.

3. Building Energy Awareness:

As the massage unfolds, cultivate awareness of energy flow within the body. Tantric philosophy recognizes the existence of subtle energy channels known as nadis or meridians. The giver can focus on stimulating and clearing these channels, fostering a balanced and heightened state of energy.

4. Exploring the Chakras:

Central to Tantric massage is the exploration of the body's energy centers, or chakras. Begin at the base and work upward, paying attention to each chakra's unique qualities. By intentionally engaging with these energy centers, the massage becomes a holistic journey that nurtures both the physical and energetic aspects of the being.

5. Yoni and Lingam Massage:

In Tantric philosophy, the yoni (vagina) and lingam (penis) are revered as sacred manifestations of divine energy. When incorporating these areas into the massage, do so with utmost respect, honoring the power and sensitivity they hold. Yoni and lingam massage can be profound sources of healing, pleasure, and connection when approached with intention and care.

6. The Dance of Polarities:

Tantric massage often involves the exploration of polarities—masculine and feminine energies, yin and yang. The giver and receiver may embody these energies in the dance of touch, creating a dynamic exchange that fosters balance and unity.

7. Awakening Sensuality:

Invite the awakening of sensuality as an integral part of the Tantric massage experience. Sensuality is not solely about physical pleasure but encompasses a heightened awareness of the senses. Engage in sensory exploration through varied textures, temperatures, and sensations to amplify the overall experience.

8. Integrating Rituals:

Consider incorporating rituals into the massage experience. This could involve the use of specific oils, candles, or symbolic gestures that align with your intentions. Rituals deepen the sense of sacredness and create a container for the transformative energies at play.

As you explore the fundamentals of Tantric massage, remember that each touch is an opportunity for connection, healing, and self-discovery. In the next chapters, we will guide you through specific techniques and practices, allowing you to integrate these fundamentals into a cohesive and enriching Tantric massage experience. May your journey be one of profound connection, awakening, and sensual exploration.

2.1 Connecting with Your Partner

Before delving into the intricate techniques of Tantric massage, it is essential to establish a deep and conscious connection with your partner. The foundation of Tantric massage lies in the energetic exchange and mutual presence between the giver and receiver. In this section, we explore the practices that foster a profound connection, setting the stage for a transformative Tantric experience.

1. Eye Contact and Presence:

Begin by establishing eye contact with your partner. Eyes are windows to the soul, and through sustained gaze, you create an immediate connection. Let your eyes convey warmth, acceptance, and a willingness to be present in this shared space. Eye contact is a powerful way to communicate without words, fostering a sense of intimacy.

2. Synchronized Breathing:

Sync your breath with your partner's. Sit facing each other and take a few moments to attune your breath to one another. Breathe in harmony, creating a shared rhythm that will serve as a foundation for the energetic exchange during the massage. Synchronized breathing deepens the connection and establishes a non-verbal communication channel.

3. Heart Center Connection:

Place your hands on each other's hearts, feeling the warmth and energy emanating from this center of love and compassion. Take a moment to connect with the heartbeat beneath your palms. This simple yet profound gesture establishes a heart-centered connection, fostering a sense of unity and shared intention.

4. Mindful Touch Exploration:

Engage in a mindful exploration of each other's bodies through gentle touch. Use your hands to trace the contours of your partner's skin, paying attention to subtle responses. This touch is not about massage techniques but rather an opportunity to attune to your partner's physical and energetic landscape.

5. Verbal Communication:

Express your intentions, desires, and boundaries through open and honest communication. Share what you hope to experience during the Tantric massage, and encourage your partner to do the same. This dialogue establishes clarity, ensuring that both participants feel heard and respected.

6. Grounding Exercise:

Sit cross-legged facing each other, with your knees touching. Rest your hands on your partner's thighs, and invite them to do the same. Close your eyes and focus on the connection between your bodies. Feel the grounding energy flowing between you, anchoring you both in the present moment.

7. Expressing Gratitude:

Take a moment to express gratitude for your partner and for the shared journey, you are about to embark upon. Verbalize your appreciation for their presence, vulnerability, and willingness to explore this sacred space with you. Gratitude sets a positive and appreciative tone for the entire experience.

8. Setting a Joint Intention:

Collaboratively decide on a joint intention for the Tantric massage. This shared purpose can be a unifying force, aligning your energies and guiding the journey. Whether it's deepening connection, exploring sensuality, or fostering healing, a joint intention amplifies the transformative potential of the experience.

Connecting with your partner in these intentional ways creates a sacred and receptive space for the Tantric massage to unfold. As you move into the subsequent sections, carry this sense of connection with you, allowing it to infuse each touch, breath, and moment of shared awareness.

2.2 Breathwork and Mindful Touch

In the intricate dance of Tantric massage, the synergy between breathwork and mindful touch serves as the heartbeat of the experience. In this section, we explore the profound connection that arises when breath and touch harmonize, elevating the massage into a sacred journey of heightened awareness and shared energy.

1. Synchronized Breathing:

Begin the Tantric massage by returning to synchronized breathing. As the giver, attune your breath to that of your partner. Create a gentle and rhythmic flow of inhalations and exhalations, fostering a shared breath that becomes the bridge connecting both your energies.

2. Breath as a Guide:

Allow the breath to guide your movements. As the giver, synchronize the pace of your touch with the rhythm of the breath. Use the inhalation to initiate a stroke and the exhalation to complete it. This mindful coordination deepens the connection and enhances the overall flow of energy.

3. Breath Awareness:

Encourage your partner to maintain awareness of their breath throughout the massage. As the receiver, focus on deep, intentional breathing. This conscious breathwork not only enhances relaxation but also amplifies the sensations and energetic exchange occurring during the massage.

4. Exploring Breath Quality:

Experiment with different qualities of breath. Invite your partner to explore slow, deep breaths, as well as quick, shallow breaths. Observe how alterations in breath impact the body's responsiveness to touch. This exploration adds a dynamic layer to the Tantric massage, allowing for a versatile and personalized experience.

5. Mindful Hand Placement:

As the giver, approach each touch with mindfulness. Let your hands become an extension of your breath, moving with intention and sensitivity. Explore varying pressures, textures, and strokes, remaining attuned to your partner's responses. Your hands become messengers of connection and presence.

6. Energetic Mapping:

Consciously map the energy of your partner's body with your hands. Feel for areas of tension, warmth, or subtle vibrations. Allow your touch to follow the natural pathways of energy flow, connecting with the body's innate wisdom. This energetic mapping deepens the sense of connection and attunement.

7. Breath Exchange:

Explore breath exchange between the giver and receiver. As the giver exhales, invite your partner to inhale, creating a cyclical exchange of breath. This practice enhances the energetic flow between you, intensifying the shared experience. Be attuned to the subtle shifts in energy that accompany this breath exchange.

8. Pause and Presence:

Incorporate moments of stillness into the massage. Pause your movements and simply rest your hands on your partner's body. Use this time for deep presence and energetic connection. These pauses allow both the giver and receiver to integrate the sensations and bask in the shared energy of the moment.

Breathwork and mindful touch are the threads that weave the fabric of Tantric massage, creating a tapestry of connection, presence, and shared energy. As you engage in these practices, remember that the essence of the experience lies not just in the physical touch, but in the dance of breath and the subtleties of energy exchange. The journey continues, inviting you to explore the depths of this sacred art.

Chapter 3: Sensual Exploration

As we venture further into the realm of Tantric massage, we enter a sacred space of sensual exploration—a journey that transcends the boundaries of mere physical touch. In this chapter, we delve into the art of heightening the senses, awakening pleasure and fostering a deep connection through the rich tapestry of Tantric sensuality.

1. Mindful Awareness:

Sensual exploration begins with mindful awareness. Both giver and receiver cultivate a heightened state of presence, allowing the senses to become acutely attuned to the nuances of touch, scent, sound, and sight. In this heightened awareness, every sensation becomes an invitation to a deeper connection.

2. Feather-Light Touch:

Experiment with a feather-light touch to evoke subtle sensations. Allow your fingertips to barely graze the skin, creating a delicate dance that tantalizes the senses. This gentle approach heightens sensitivity and fosters a profound awareness of the body's responsiveness.

3. Varying Textures:

Introduce an array of textures during the massage. Silky fabrics, warm oils, and cool stones can add layers to the sensory experience. The juxtaposition of textures awakens different sensory receptors, amplifying the pleasure and expanding the scope of the sensual journey.

4. Aromatherapy and Scents:

Incorporate the power of aromatherapy to stimulate the olfactory senses. Essential oils like jasmine, sandalwood, or rose can evoke feelings of sensuality and relaxation. The subtle interplay of scents contributes to the overall ambiance, creating a multi-dimensional sensory experience.

5. Soundscapes:

Select a curated soundtrack or ambient soundscape to enhance the auditory dimension of the experience. The gentle rustle of leaves, the soothing flow of water, or melodic tunes can create a harmonious backdrop, resonating with the energies of the Tantric massage.

6. Temperature Play:

Explore the element of temperature to add a layer of excitement to the massage. Warm oils, cool stones, or even heated towels can introduce pleasurable sensations. Temperature play not only stimulates the skin but also creates a dynamic and immersive sensory experience.

7. Sensual Breathwork:

Incorporate intentional breathing to amplify sensuality. Encourage your partner to breathe deeply and audibly, allowing the breath to become a sensual soundtrack. Sync your breath with theirs, creating a rhythm that harmonizes with the ebb and flow of the massage.

8. Heightening Erotic Energy:

As the massage progresses, explore the intentional awakening of erotic energy. This is not about performance but about acknowledging and celebrating the body's capacity for pleasure. Cultivate a space where both giver and receiver feel safe expressing and embracing their sensual selves.

9. Sacred Union of Hearts:

Deepen the connection by bringing a sense of sacredness to the union of hearts. Encourage heart-centered touch, allowing the hands to rest over the heart center. This gentle connection fosters an emotional intimacy that transcends the physical, creating a profound and sacred space.

In the exploration of sensuality, Tantric massage becomes a symphony of the senses, inviting participants to immerse themselves in the richness of the present moment. As you engage in this chapter's practices, remember that the true essence of sensuality lies in the mindful celebration of the body, the senses, and the shared journey of intimate connection. The

Tantric odyssey continues, weaving together the threads of touch, breath, and profound awareness.

3.1 Awakening the Senses

In the intricate tapestry of Tantric massage, the art of sensual exploration begins with a conscious awakening of the senses. This section delves into practices designed to heighten awareness, stimulate pleasure, and create a sensory symphony that transcends the ordinary, ushering participants into a realm of heightened intimacy.

1. Mindful Grounding:

Commence the sensual journey with a grounding practice. Sit in a comfortable position, and together with your partner, focus on your breath. Inhale deeply, drawing energy from the earth, and exhale, releasing any tension or distractions. This practice establishes a centered foundation for the sensual exploration that follows.

2. Sensory Meditation:

Engage in a sensory meditation to attune your awareness. With closed eyes, take turns describing sensations that each sense perceives. Share the touch of the air, the rustle of fabric, or the scent of the surroundings. This exercise deepens present-moment awareness and opens the door to a heightened sensual experience.

3. Feather-Light Exploration:

Begin the Tantric massage with a feather-light touch. Utilize soft strokes and delicate caresses, exploring the contours of your partner's body with exquisite gentleness. This subtle touch initiates a dance of sensitivity, inviting the receiver into a realm of heightened tactile awareness.

4. Blindfold Sensory Adventure:

Introduce an element of anticipation and mystery by incorporating a blindfold. As the receiver, being blindfolded enhances other senses, intensifying the experience of touch, scent, and sound. The giver, in turn, becomes attuned to the subtleties of their partner's responses, creating a dynamic exchange of energies.

5. Scented Oils and Aromas:

Select scented oils or aromas to enrich the olfactory experience. As the giver, infuse the massage space with fragrances that evoke sensuality and relaxation. Explore the delightful interplay of scents, allowing the aroma to become an integral part of the sensory landscape.

6. Temperature Contrast:

Engage in temperature play to stimulate the sense of touch. Alternating between warm and cool sensations creates a dynamic and pleasurable experience. Consider using warm oils or cool stones to awaken different areas of the body, heightening the overall sensory exploration.

7. Sound Resonance:

Integrate intentional sounds to resonate with the auditory senses. Gentle music, whispers, or synchronized breaths contribute to a melodic backdrop that enhances the atmosphere. The rhythmic harmony of sound creates a sensual symphony, inviting participants into a deeper state of connection.

8. Taste Sensations:

Incorporate taste into the sensory exploration. Experiment with the subtle taste of fruits, chocolates, or other edible delights. As the receiver, savor each moment, allowing the sense of taste to enhance the overall pleasure and connection.

9. Mindful Sensual Pause:

Periodically pause during the massage to engage in mindful sensory awareness. Encourage your partner to become fully present in the sensations arising from touch, scent, sound, and taste. These pauses serve as anchors, deepening the connection and allowing the experience to unfold organically.

Awakening the senses is a gateway to a profound Tantric exploration. By engaging in these practices, participants embark on a journey that transcends the ordinary, weaving together the threads of touch, breath, and heightened awareness. As you move through this chapter, let the awakening of the senses be a conscious celebration of the body, a sacred dance of intimacy, and an invitation to deeper connection.

3.2 Building Trust and Communication

In the intricate dance of Tantric massage, trust and communication form the sturdy foundation upon which the transformative journey unfolds. This section explores the essential practices and principles that build a space of trust, vulnerability, and open communication—key elements in fostering a profound and connected Tantric experience.

1. Creating a Safe Space:

Establishing a safe space is paramount in building trust. Ensure that the physical environment is comfortable, private, and free from external disturbances. Cultivate an atmosphere where both giver and receiver feel secure in expressing their needs, desires, and boundaries.

2. Open Dialogue:

Encourage open dialogue before, during, and after the Tantric massage. Before the session, discuss intentions, expectations, and any concerns that may arise. During the massage, maintain a continuous exchange of verbal and non-verbal communication to ensure both participants feel heard and respected.

3. Non-verbal Cues:

Develop an understanding of non-verbal cues. Create a system of signals or gestures that allow the receiver to communicate their comfort level during the massage. Whether it's a subtle hand movement or a predetermined signal, non-verbal communication enhances the flow of trust and understanding.

4. Active Listening:

Practice active listening as an integral part of communication. Both giver and receiver should be attuned to verbal and non-verbal cues, acknowledging and responding to each other's expressions. Active listening creates a responsive and empathetic connection, fostering a deeper level of trust.

5. Expressing Boundaries:

Establish clear boundaries and encourage their open expression. As the giver, check in with your partner regularly to ensure they feel comfortable and respected. The receiver, in turn, is empowered to communicate any shifts in comfort, allowing both participants to navigate the experience with trust and mutual understanding.

6. Consent and Permission:

Prioritize the importance of explicit consent and permission. Any new technique, exploration, or shift in intensity should be communicated and agreed upon by both participants. Establishing a culture of consent enhances trust and ensures that the boundaries of each participant are honored.

7. Trust-Building Rituals:

Incorporate trust-building rituals into the Tantric massage experience. This could involve a shared meditation, a moment of eye contact, or a simple touch that symbolizes the commitment to mutual trust. These rituals deepen the sense of connection and create a foundation of trust for the journey ahead.

8. Aftercare and Debriefing:

Allocate time for aftercare and debriefing following the Tantric massage. Engage in a reflective conversation where both giver and receiver share their experiences, feelings, and insights. This post-massage dialogue not only deepens the connection but also establishes a supportive space for processing the journey.

9. Emotional Vulnerability:

Recognize and honor the potential for emotional vulnerability that may arise during the Tantric massage. Encourage an atmosphere where both participants feel safe expressing and exploring their emotions. Emotional openness deepens the connection and allows for a more profound and transformative experience.

Building trust and communication transforms Tantric massage from a physical exchange into a sacred and emotionally resonant journey. As you engage in these practices, may the space you create be one of openness, respect, and shared vulnerability—an environment where trust blossoms and the transformative potential of Tantric massage unfolds.

Chapter 4: Techniques for Beginners

Embarking on the path of Tantric massage is a journey into the art of sensual connection and mindful touch. In this chapter, we explore foundational techniques that cater to beginners, providing a practical guide to initiate the dance of energy, pleasure, and intimacy. Whether you are a giver or a receiver, these techniques are designed to foster a harmonious and transformative Tantric experience.

1. **Conscious Touch:**

The essence of Tantric massage lies in conscious touch. Begin by placing your hands on your partner's body with awareness and intention. Allow your touch to be exploratory, gentle, and mindful. Feel the energy exchange between your hands and your partner's skin, creating a connection that goes beyond the physical.

2. **Effleurage Strokes:**

Effleurage strokes are long, gliding movements that serve as a warm-up for the massage. Using the entire surface of your hands, move rhythmically over your partner's body. This technique promotes relaxation, stimulates blood circulation, and establishes a sense of comfort and trust.

3. Feathering Technique:

Introduce the feathering technique for a delicate and sensual touch. Lightly trace your fingertips over your partner's skin, creating a subtle sensation. This technique is designed to awaken the skin's sensitivity, heightening awareness and paving the way for deeper exploration.

4. Kneading Motion:

Incorporate the kneading motion to release tension in specific areas. Use your hands to gently lift, squeeze, and release the muscles. This technique promotes relaxation, eases muscular tightness, and encourages the flow of energy through the body.

5. Circular Thumb Movements:

Focus on circular thumb movements to target specific points of tension. Use your thumbs to create small, circular motions on areas like the shoulders, neck, or lower back. Adjust the pressure based on your partner's comfort, allowing the thumbs to penetrate and release tension.

6. Yoni and Lingam Massage Basics:

For those comfortable exploring intimate areas, introduce the basics of Yoni (vagina) and Lingam (penis) massage. Approach these areas with utmost respect and communicate openly. Use gentle, circular motions and varying pressures to create a space of pleasure, healing, and connection.

7.   Balancing Energy Centers (Chakras):

Explore the balancing of energy centers, or chakras, during the massage. Place your hands over each chakra, starting from the base of the spine and moving upward. Focus on creating a sense of warmth and energy flow, allowing your touch to harmonize and balance the subtle energies within the body.

8.   Breathwork Integration:

Integrate intentional breathwork into the massage experience. Encourage synchronized breathing between you and your partner. Let the rhythm of the breath guide your movements, enhancing the energetic connection and deepening the overall sense of intimacy.

9.   Dynamic Feedback:

Maintain dynamic feedback throughout the massage. As the giver, observe your partner's responses and adjust your techniques accordingly. Encourage the receiver to communicate their preferences and comfort levels, fostering a continuous dialogue that enriches the shared experience.

10. Closing Ritual:

Conclude the Tantric massage with a closing ritual. This could involve a moment of shared breath, a gentle embrace, or a few moments of quiet connection. The closing ritual serves as a transition, allowing both the giver and receiver to integrate the experience and express gratitude for the shared journey.

As you explore these techniques, remember that Tantric massage is an evolving practice that unfolds uniquely for each participant. Approach the journey with an open heart, a willingness to learn, and a commitment to the sacred exchange of energy and connection. May this chapter be a guide for beginners, illuminating the path toward a more profound and enriching Tantric experience.

4.1 Basic Massage Strokes

As you embark on the journey of Tantric massage, mastering basic massage strokes lays the foundation for a harmonious and connected experience. In this section, we delve into fundamental techniques that form the backbone of Tantric touch, fostering relaxation, sensitivity, and a deeper connection between the giver and the receiver.

1. **Effleurage Strokes:**

Effleurage, or gliding strokes, serve as a gentle introduction to the massage. Using the entire surface of your hands, create long, rhythmic strokes along your partner's body. This technique promotes relaxation, warms the muscles, and establishes a sense of trust and comfort.

2. **Petrissage Technique:**

Petrissage involves kneading movements that target specific muscle groups. Use your hands to lift and squeeze the muscles gently, applying varying pressures. This technique is effective in releasing tension, enhancing circulation, and preparing the body for a more focused touch.

3. **Circular Friction:**

Circular friction involves small, circular movements with your fingertips or thumbs. Apply this technique to specific areas with tension or knots, using a comfortable amount of pressure. Circular friction stimulates blood flow, relieves localized tension, and encourages a sense of release.

4. **Tapotement (Rhythmic Tapping):**

Tapotement is a percussive technique involving rhythmic tapping or drumming motions. Use cupped hands or fingertips to lightly tap or pat the surface of your partner's skin. This invigorating technique helps awaken the senses, increase circulation, and enliven the body.

5.   Feathering Strokes:

Feathering strokes involve using the lightest touch, like the caress of a feather, to awaken the skin's sensitivity. Trace your fingertips delicately over your partner's body, creating a subtle and sensuous experience. Feathering strokes prepare the body for a more focused and intimate touch.

6.   Stretching Movements:

Incorporate gentle stretching movements into the massage to increase flexibility and release tension. Gradually stretch limbs, moving joints through their natural range of motion. This technique promotes relaxation, enhances body awareness, and encourages a deeper connection between the giver and receiver.

7.   Compression Technique:

Compression involves applying sustained pressure to specific points using your palms, thumbs, or elbows. This technique can be used to release tension in muscles and trigger points. Adjust the pressure based on your partner's comfort, allowing for a gradual release of muscular tightness.

8.   Balancing Energy Centers (Chakras):

Focus on balancing energy centers, or chakras, through light touch and intention. Place your hands over each chakra, starting from the base of the spine and moving upward. Feel the energy beneath your hands, and use gentle circular motions to harmonize and balance the subtle energies within the body.

9.   Sensual Stroking:

Introduce sensual stroking to enhance the intimate connection between the giver and receiver. Use the entire surface of your hands to create slow, deliberate strokes that explore the contours of your partner's body. Sensual stroking fosters a deeper sense of intimacy and connection.

10. Joint Mobilization:

Incorporate joint mobilization to improve joint flexibility and release tension. Gently move joints through their natural range of motion, paying attention to the comfort level of your partner. Joint mobilization adds a therapeutic element to the massage, promoting overall well-being.

As you practice these basic massage strokes, remember that Tantric massage is a shared journey of exploration and connection. Focus on being present, responsive to your partner's cues, and open to the transformative potential of touch. With these foundational techniques, may your Tantric massage experience unfold as a sacred dance of energy and intimacy.

4.2 Exploring Erotic Zones

In the realm of Tantric massage, the exploration of erotic zones adds a layer of intimacy and pleasure to the shared experience. In this section, we delve into techniques for respectfully and sensually exploring areas of heightened sensitivity, fostering a deeper connection, and awakening the body's capacity for pleasure.

1. **Communication and Consent:**

Before venturing into the exploration of erotic zones, establish open communication and obtain clear consent from your partner. Create a space where both giver and receiver feel empowered to express their desires, boundaries, and comfort levels. Consensual exploration is key to a mutually enriching experience.

2. **Feather-Light Touch:**

Initiate the exploration with a feather-light touch. Use gentle strokes and caresses to trace the contours of areas considered erotic zones. The lightness of touch serves to heighten sensitivity and build anticipation, creating a delicate and intimate connection.

3.   Nurturing the Neck and Ears:

The neck and ears are potent erogenous zones. Employ gentle kisses, nibbles, or soft breaths to stimulate these areas. Incorporate light massage and explore the sensitivity of the skin, allowing your touch to evoke both relaxation and a subtle awakening of erotic energy.

4.   Sensual Stroking Along the Spine:

The spine is an energetically rich area that, when sensually stroked, can evoke pleasurable sensations. Use long, slow strokes along the spine, paying attention to the entire length of the back. This technique not only relaxes the muscles but also creates a pathway for the flow of sensual energy.

5.   Intimate Touch on the Inner Thighs:

The inner thighs are highly sensitive and responsive to touch. With gentleness and respect, explore this area using feathering strokes, light kisses, or subtle caresses. Be attuned to your partner's comfort level, and communicate openly as you venture into this intimate territory.

6. Abdominal Awakening:

The abdominal region holds a unique blend of vulnerability and sensuality. Employ light circular motions with your fingertips, exploring the contours of the abdomen. This technique invites a connection with the sacral chakra, fostering pleasure and awakening erotic energy within the body.

7. Yoni and Lingam Exploration:

For those comfortable with intimate exploration, introduce the basics of Yoni (vagina) and Lingam (penis) massage. Approach these areas with profound respect, acknowledging their sacredness. Utilize gentle, intentional touch, exploring the diverse sensations and fostering a space for healing, pleasure, and connection.

8. Mindful Exploration of Hands and Feet:

Hands and feet contain numerous nerve endings, making them zones of heightened sensitivity. Apply mindful exploration, using gentle massage, circular motions, or feather-light touch on the palms, fingers, soles, and toes. This technique amplifies overall sensitivity and stimulates pleasurable sensations.

9.   Guided Breathwork for Sensual Connection:

Integrate guided breathwork into the exploration of erotic zones. Encourage synchronized breathing between the giver and receiver, creating a rhythmic exchange of energy. Breathwork enhances the connection, heightening the sensual experience and promoting a shared journey of pleasure.

10. Closing Ritual and Reflection:

Conclude the exploration of erotic zones with a closing ritual that acknowledges the sacredness of the shared experience. Engage in a moment of shared breath, a gentle embrace, or verbal expressions of gratitude. Encourage open reflection on the experience, fostering a sense of connection and mutual understanding.

Remember that the exploration of erotic zones in Tantric massage is a collaborative journey that demands sensitivity, communication, and respect. Approach each touch with mindfulness, prioritize consent, and create an atmosphere of shared vulnerability and pleasure. In the dance of energy and intimacy, may the exploration of erotic zones deepen your connection and enrich the sacred tapestry of Tantric massage.

Chapter 5: Deepening Intimacy

In the profound landscape of Tantric massage, the journey of deepening intimacy unfolds as a sacred dance between the giver and the receiver. This chapter explores advanced techniques and practices designed to foster a heightened sense of connection, trust, and profound intimacy. Whether you are a seasoned practitioner or exploring Tantric massage for the first time, these advanced strategies invite you to delve into the depths of sacred connection and shared vulnerability.

1.   **Tantric Breath Fusion:**

Elevate the connection between giver and receiver by engaging in Tantric breath fusion. In a synchronized and intentional manner, let your breaths become one. As you inhale and exhale together, the shared breath creates a profound energetic exchange, deepening the sense of oneness and intimacy.

2.   **Extended Eye Gazing:**

Incorporate extended periods of eye gazing into the Tantric massage experience. As the giver and receiver lock eyes, allow a deep soul connection to unfold. Eye gazing creates a gateway to the essence of each other, fostering a level of intimacy that transcends words and physical touch.

3. Energy Mapping Meditation:

Before the massage, engage in an energy-mapping meditation. As the giver, visualize and feel the flow of energy within your own body. Extend this awareness to your partner, sensing their energetic landscape. This practice enhances sensitivity, deepening the connection during the massage.

4. Mutual Heart Connection:

Establish a mutual heart connection between the giver and the receiver. Place your hands over each other's hearts and synchronize your breaths. Feel the energetic exchange between the heart centers, fostering a shared space of love, compassion, and emotional intimacy.

5. Sacred Mantras and Affirmations:

Integrate sacred mantras or affirmations into the massage experience. As you touch and connect, speak words of love, healing, and affirmation. The power of spoken intention amplifies the energetic resonance, deepening the transformative potential of the Tantric journey.

6. Subtle Energetic Bonding:

Explore subtle energetic bonding through intentional touch and visualization. As the giver, imagine a thread of golden light connecting your heart to your partner's heart. With each touch, visualize energy flowing through this connection, creating a bond that transcends the physical realm.

7. Ritualistic Anointing:

Incorporate a ritualistic anointing ceremony using sacred oils. As the giver anoints the receiver, consider the symbolic significance of this act. The anointing ritual serves as a consecration, infusing the massage with a sense of sanctity and deepening the overall sacred connection.

8. Shared Mindful Meditation:

Before the massage, engage in a shared mindful meditation. Sit together, focus on your breath, and create a shared space of presence. This meditation deepens the connection and attunement between giver and receiver, aligning energies and setting the stage for a profound Tantric experience.

9.   Integrating Sound Healing:

Explore the use of sound healing instruments or vocal toning during the massage. Harmonious sounds, whether from singing bowls, chimes, or the human voice, can amplify the energetic resonance, creating a vibrational symphony that deepens the sense of connection and intimacy.

10. Unspoken Sensual Language:

Cultivate an unspoken sensual language during the massage. Let your hands convey emotions, desires, and intentions without the need for verbal communication. This intuitive exchange fosters a level of intimacy that transcends language, allowing the energy to speak for itself.

As you embark on the journey of deepening intimacy in Tantric massage, approach each practice with reverence, openness, and a commitment to shared exploration. In the dance of energy and connection, may this chapter guide you toward the sacred depths of Tantric intimacy, where the transformative power of touch unfolds in its most profound and transcendent forms.

5.1 Emotional Connection

In the sacred realm of Tantric massage, the exploration of emotional connection adds a profound dimension to the shared journey of intimacy. This section delves into advanced practices and techniques designed to deepen the emotional bond between the giver and the receiver. By cultivating a space of vulnerability, trust, and open-hearted communication, the Tantric massage becomes a transformative vessel for emotional connection.

1.   Heart-Centered Meditation:

Commence the Tantric massage experience with a heart-centered meditation. As both giver and receiver, bring awareness to the heart center and synchronize your breaths. Allow the meditation to create a harmonious space where emotions can be felt and expressed, fostering a deep emotional connection.

2.   Emotional Check-In:

Prioritize emotional well-being by initiating an emotional check-in before the massage. The giver and receiver openly share their current emotional states, expressing any feelings or concerns. This practice establishes an atmosphere of emotional awareness, promoting a more attuned and supportive connection.

3.   Energetic Emotional Release:

Incorporate energetic emotional release techniques into the massage. As the giver, use intuitive touch to explore areas of tension or holding within the body. Encourage the receiver to express emotions that may arise, allowing the massage to serve as a cathartic release of stored energy and emotions.

4. Witnessing and Mirroring:

Practice the art of witnessing and mirroring emotions during the massage. The giver and receiver take turns acknowledging and verbalizing the emotions that arise. This reflective dialogue creates a safe space for emotional expression and deepens the connection through shared vulnerability.

5. Emotional Breathwork:

Engage in emotional breathwork as a dynamic component of the Tantric massage. Encourage the receiver to breathe into and express their emotions through audible breaths. The rhythmic exchange of breath becomes a vehicle for emotional release and a conduit for shared energy and connection.

6. Healing Touch for Emotional Release:

Utilize a healing touch to facilitate emotional release. Gently place your hands on areas where emotional tension is stored, allowing the energy to be acknowledged and released through touch. This technique honors the emotional landscape, creating a transformative and nurturing experience.

7.   Integration of Affirmations:

Integrate positive affirmations into the massage, focusing on emotional well-being. Use spoken words to affirm feelings of love, acceptance, and safety. Affirmations create a supportive environment, allowing emotions to be expressed and embraced with compassion.

8.   Embracing Tears:

Recognize and honor the potential for tears as a form of emotional release. As tears flow, maintain a space of compassion and acceptance. Allow the tears to be a natural expression of emotions, fostering a sense of liberation and healing within the intimate connection.

9.   Shared Emotional Intentions:

Co-create shared emotional intentions for the Tantric massage experience. Verbally express the emotions you both wish to cultivate during the session, such as love, joy, or serenity. These shared intentions serve as a guiding force, shaping the emotional landscape of the massage.

10. Post-Massage Emotional Integration:

Allocate time for post-massage emotional integration. Engage in a reflective conversation where the giver and receiver share their emotional experiences and insights. This dialogue creates a sense of closure, allowing both participants to integrate the emotional aspects of the Tantric journey.

In the exploration of emotional connection within Tantric massage, authenticity, and open-heartedness become the guiding principles. As you engage in these advanced practices, may the emotional tapestry woven during the massage deepen the connection between giver and receiver, fostering a transformative and heart-centered experience.

5.2 Nurturing Intimacy beyond the Massage

The essence of Tantric massage extends beyond the confines of the massage session, permeating into the fabric of daily life. This section explores advanced strategies for nurturing intimacy beyond the massage, fostering a sustained and profound connection between the giver and the receiver. By incorporating mindful practices and intentional gestures, the transformative power of Tantric intimacy becomes a continuous thread woven into the tapestry of your relationship.

1. **Sacred Rituals of Connection:**

Introduce sacred rituals of connection that extend beyond the massage setting. These rituals may include shared meditation, candlelit moments, or simply expressing gratitude for each other. Sacred rituals create a consistent space for connection, infusing everyday life with the sacred energy cultivated during Tantric massage.

2.   Daily Mindful Touch:

Incorporate daily mindful touch into your routine. Giver and receiver can engage in brief moments of intentional touch—a hand on the heart, a gentle caress, or a lingering hug. These moments of connection serve as reminders of the deep intimacy experienced during Tantric massage, weaving the energy of touch into daily life.

3.   Heart-Centered Communication:

Cultivate heart-centered communication in your interactions. Embrace open and vulnerable conversations, sharing your thoughts, feelings, and desires with authenticity. This level of communication deepens emotional intimacy, creating a foundation for sustained connection beyond the realms of the Tantric massage.

4.   Mutual Exploration of Desires:

Engage in a mutual exploration of desires and fantasies. Create a safe space where both partners feel empowered to express their intimate desires. This open dialogue fosters a sense of shared vulnerability and deepens the understanding of each other's needs, strengthening the intimate connection.

5.   Collaborative Breathwork Practices:

Explore collaborative breathwork practices during moments of connection. Engage in synchronized breathing, allowing your breaths to harmonize. Breathwork serves as a continuous bridge between giver and receiver, fostering an ongoing connection that transcends the boundaries of time and space.

6.   Sensory Enrichment in Shared Spaces:

Enhance shared spaces with sensory elements. Introduce soft lighting, soothing scents, and tactile textures to create an environment that nurtures intimacy. These sensory-rich spaces serve as a backdrop for moments of connection, enveloping you both in the energy cultivated during Tantric massage.

7.   Mindful Presence in Daily Interactions:

Infuse mindful presence into your daily interactions. Whether cooking together, engaging in a shared activity, or simply spending time in each other's company, practice being fully present. Mindful presence deepens the sense of connection and allows the energy of intimacy to permeate ordinary moments.

8.   Expressing Gratitude:

Make expressing gratitude a daily practice. Take moments to acknowledge and appreciate each other's presence, kindness, and love. Gratitude becomes a powerful force, amplifying the positive energy within the relationship and reinforcing the emotional and intimate connection.

9.   Shared Spiritual Practices:

Explore shared spiritual practices that resonate with both partners. This may include meditation, prayer, or any form of spiritual connection. Engaging in shared spiritual practices deepens the sense of unity and provides a sacred foundation for the ongoing journey of intimacy.

10.   Regular Check-Ins:

Incorporate regular check-ins into your relationship routine. These check-ins serve as dedicated moments to discuss your emotional states, desires, and any adjustments needed in your intimate connection. This ongoing dialogue ensures that the bond forged during Tantric massage continues to evolve and thrive.

As you embrace the practice of nurturing intimacy beyond the Tantric massage, may your relationship become a sanctuary where the transformative energy of touch, connection, and love is woven into the very fabric of your shared existence. Through these advanced strategies, may the journey of Tantric intimacy extend its embrace into the richness of your everyday life.

Chapter 6: Overcoming Challenges

Embarking on the path of Tantric massage is a transformative journey, but like any profound exploration, it may come with its set of challenges. This chapter addresses common obstacles that may arise during the practice of Tantric massage and offers guidance on how to navigate these challenges. By acknowledging and understanding these hurdles, you can empower yourself and your partner to overcome them, fostering a deeper and more enriching Tantric experience.

1. **Communication Breakdown:**

Challenge: Breakdowns in communication can hinder the flow of energy and intimacy during Tantric massage.

Solution: Prioritize open and honest communication. Establish a non-judgmental space where both giver and receiver feel comfortable expressing their needs, desires, and concerns. Regular check-ins before, during, and after the massage can enhance communication and deepen understanding.

2.   Expectation Misalignment:

Challenge: Divergent expectations between the giver and receiver may lead to misunderstandings or disappointment.

Solution: Initiate a dialogue to align expectations before each Tantric massage session. Discuss intentions, boundaries, and any preferences to ensure that both partners are on the same page. Flexibility and a willingness to adapt to each other's needs contribute to a more harmonious experience.

3.   Discomfort with Vulnerability:

Challenge: The practice of Tantric massage involves a level of vulnerability that may be uncomfortable for some individuals.

Solution: Foster a supportive and non-judgmental environment that encourages vulnerability. Engage in heart-centered conversations, affirm the sacred nature of the experience, and emphasize the mutual trust between the giver and the receiver. Gradual exploration and reassurance can help ease discomfort.

4.   Emotional Release Overwhelm:

Challenge: Intense emotional releases, such as tears or unexpected emotions, may overwhelm either the giver or the receiver.

Solution: Establish a foundation of emotional safety and acceptance. Encourage open expression of emotions and reassure both partners that such releases are natural and welcomed. Create a plan for post-massage debriefing to process and integrate any intense emotional experiences.

5. Time Constraints:

Challenge: Limited time for Tantric massage sessions may hinder the depth of connection and exploration.

Solution: Prioritize quality over quantity. If time is a constraint, focus on creating intentional and mindful moments during shorter sessions. Set realistic expectations and use the time available to deepen specific aspects of the Tantric experience.

6. Physical Discomfort or Pain:

Challenge: Physical discomfort or pain during the massage can detract from the overall experience.

Solution: Establish clear communication about physical sensations. Encourage the receiver to express any discomfort or pain, and adjust techniques accordingly. Use variations in pressure, explore alternative techniques, and prioritize the well-being and comfort of both partners.

7.   **Distractions and External Factors:**

Challenge: External distractions or environmental factors may disrupt the Tantric experience.

Solution: Create a dedicated and serene space for Tantric massage, minimizing potential distractions. Set the intention to create a sacred atmosphere and discuss any external factors that may affect the experience. Silence phones, dim lights, and create an environment conducive to focused connection.

8.   **Resistance to Change:**

Challenge: Resistance to change or trying new practices may surface, hindering the exploration of Tantric techniques.

Solution: Approach Tantric massage with an open mind and a spirit of curiosity. Encourage a sense of playfulness and exploration. Acknowledge any resistance and communicate openly about feelings or concerns. Gradual introduction and mutual consent facilitate a more comfortable embrace of new practices.

9.   **Personal Insecurities:**

Challenge: Personal insecurities, body image concerns, or self-judgment may arise.

Solution: Foster a space of acceptance and appreciation. Encourage positive affirmations, both internally and verbally. Emphasize the beauty of vulnerability and the shared experience. Mutual reassurance and genuine compliments can help dispel personal insecurities, allowing for a more liberated and connected experience.

10. Post-Massage Integration:

Challenge: Difficulty in integrating the Tantric experience into daily life may hinder its long-term impact.

Solution: Establish post-massage rituals or reflections that facilitate integration. Engage in shared activities, discussions, or moments of gratitude after the session. Encourage ongoing communication about the effects and insights gained from Tantric massage, reinforcing its transformative potential.

By addressing and navigating these challenges with sensitivity and openness, you and your partner can cultivate a resilient and fulfilling Tantric practice. Embrace the journey, celebrate the shared discoveries, and view challenges as opportunities for growth and deeper connection. Through mindful navigation, may the challenges encountered become stepping stones towards a more profound and enriching Tantric experience.

6.1 Addressing Discomfort

In the intricate dance of Tantric massage, moments of discomfort may arise, disrupting the flow of connection and energy. It is essential to approach these instances with sensitivity and a commitment to maintaining a safe and nurturing space. This section guides addressing discomfort, ensuring that both giver and receiver can navigate challenges and continue their Tantric journey with openness and understanding.

1.   **Open Communication:**

Encourage open and honest communication as the cornerstone for addressing discomfort. Establish a verbal and non-verbal dialogue that allows both partners to express their feelings, sensations, and concerns without judgment. This creates a foundation for understanding and mutual support.

2.   **Gentle Check-Ins:**

Incorporate gentle check-ins throughout the Tantric massage session. As the giver, periodically ask the receiver about their comfort level, ensuring that the pace and intensity align with their preferences. Establishing a continuous feedback loop fosters a sense of trust and allows for adjustments in real time.

3.   **Empowerment Through Choice:**

Empower the receiver by offering choices. Provide options for different techniques, pressures, or areas of focus. This empowers the receiver to actively participate in shaping the massage experience, fostering a sense of control and comfort over their journey.

4.   Mindful Technique Adjustments:

As the giver, remain attuned to the receiver's body language and verbal cues. If discomfort is detected, be prepared to adjust your techniques. Modify pressure, change the rhythm of movements, or explore alternative approaches to ensure a more comfortable and enjoyable experience.

5.   Exploration of Boundaries:

Encourage open exploration of boundaries. Discuss any physical or emotional boundaries before the massage and create an atmosphere where both partners feel safe expressing their limits. Respecting and acknowledging boundaries is crucial for maintaining a sense of security and trust.

6.   Breathing Through Discomfort:

Guide the receiver in using intentional breathwork to navigate discomfort. Encourage deep, rhythmic breathing to promote relaxation and release tension. Breathwork serves as a powerful tool for both the giver and receiver to manage sensations and foster a deeper connection with the present moment.

7.   Emotional Validation:

Acknowledge and validate any emotions that arise with discomfort. Create a space where the receiver feels supported in expressing their feelings. Emotional validation fosters a sense of understanding and empathy, allowing both partners to navigate discomfort with compassion.

8.   Gradual Exploration:

Approach Tantric techniques with a gradual and exploratory mindset. Introduce new practices incrementally, allowing the receiver to acclimate to different sensations. Gradual exploration promotes a sense of comfort, reducing the likelihood of overwhelming discomfort during the session.

9.   Adjusting Environmental Factors:

Evaluate and adjust environmental factors that may contribute to discomfort. Ensure the room temperature is comfortable, minimize external distractions, and create an ambiance that promotes relaxation. A harmonious environment enhances the overall sense of well-being during Tantric massage.

10. Post-Massage Debriefing:

Allocate time for post-massage debriefing to address any lingering discomfort. Engage in a reflective conversation where both giver and receiver share their experiences, concerns, and insights. This debriefing process provides closure and supports the integration of the Tantric journey.

By incorporating these approaches, discomfort within the realm of Tantric massage can be acknowledged, understood, and transformed into an opportunity for growth and deeper connection. With compassion, communication, and a shared commitment to mutual well-being, the Tantric experience can continue to unfold as a sacred and transformative journey.

6.2 Communication during the Practice

Effective communication is the heartbeat of a profound Tantric massage experience, fostering connection, understanding, and a harmonious flow of energy. In this section, we delve into the importance of communication during the practice, guiding both giver and receiver to engage in a dialogue that enhances the overall depth and transformative potential of the Tantric journey.

1. **Establishing Verbal and Non-Verbal Cues:**

Create a language of communication that combines both verbal and non-verbal cues. While words convey explicit messages, non-verbal signals such as sighs, breathe patterns, or subtle movements can provide additional insights into the receiver's experience. Establishing a comprehensive communication framework enriches the connection between partners.

2. **Continuous Check-Ins:**

Integrate continuous check-ins throughout the Tantric massage session. As the giver, inquire about the receiver's comfort, preferences, and sensations. Encourage the receiver to express their feelings and provide feedback. This ongoing dialogue ensures that the massage experience is co-created and responsive to the evolving needs of both partners.

3. **Encouraging Feedback:**

Cultivate an atmosphere that encourages honest and constructive feedback. Both giver and receiver should feel empowered to express their experiences, preferences, and any adjustments they may require. Open dialogue enriches the mutual understanding of desires, fostering a collaborative and co-creative Tantric experience.

4. **Non-Judgmental Listening:**

Practice non-judgmental listening to truly hear and understand your partner. As the giver, be attuned to verbal cues and body language, offering a space where the receiver feels heard and acknowledged. Non-judgmental listening fosters trust and strengthens the emotional connection during the Tantric massage.

5.   Mutual Intentions Discussion:

Initiate a discussion about mutual intentions before the practice begins. Both partners can share their desires, expectations, and any boundaries they wish to establish. Aligning intentions sets the foundation for a shared understanding, reducing the likelihood of miscommunication and enhancing the overall Tantric experience.

6.   Language of Sensations:

Explore a language of sensations to articulate experiences that go beyond words. Encourage the receiver to describe the quality of touch, the intensity of sensations, and the emotions elicited during the massage. This expressive use of language deepens the connection and allows for a more nuanced understanding of the Tantric journey.

7.   Synchronized Breathing:

Integrate synchronized breathing as a form of communication. Coordinate your breath with your partner's, creating a rhythmic exchange that enhances energetic connection. Shared breathwork serves as a silent yet powerful means of communication, facilitating a synchronized and harmonious Tantric experience.

8.   Gentle Guidance and Permission Seeking:

As the giver, provide gentle guidance during the massage and seek permission before exploring new techniques or areas of focus. This ensures that both partners feel respected and in control of the experience. Permission-seeking fosters a collaborative approach to the Tantric practice.

9.   Empathy and Validation:

Cultivate empathy and validation in your communication. Acknowledge and validate your partner's experiences, feelings, and expressions. This creates a supportive space where both the giver and receiver feel understood, fostering emotional intimacy and trust.

10.   Post-Massage Reflection:

Allocate time for post-massage reflection and discussion. Share your thoughts, insights, and emotions in a reflective conversation. This post-massage dialogue allows for the integration of the Tantric experience and provides an opportunity for partners to deepen their connection through shared reflection.

By prioritizing communication during the Tantric massage practice, partners can co-create a transformative and enriching experience. Through attentive listening, open dialogue, and a shared commitment to understanding each other's needs, the Tantric journey becomes a sacred and harmonious exchange of energy and intimacy.

Chapter 7: Advanced Practices

In the expansive realm of Tantric massage, advanced practices beckon those who seek to delve deeper into the sacred art of sensual connection and spiritual exploration. This chapter unfolds a tapestry of advanced techniques, rituals, and approaches that elevate the Tantric experience to new heights. Whether you are a seasoned practitioner or venturing into advanced practices for the first time, these offerings invite you to embark on a journey of profound intimacy and transformation.

1. Tantric Connection Ritual:

Begin your Tantric massage session with a dedicated connection ritual. Engage in synchronized breathwork, mutual eye gazing, and gentle touches to align energies. This ritual establishes a sacred container, inviting a deep connection between the giver and receiver before the more intricate practices unfold.

2. Chakra Balancing Massage:

Explore the ancient wisdom of the chakras by incorporating a chakra-balancing massage. Focus on each energy center, using intentional touch and energy awareness to harmonize and activate these vital points. This practice enhances energetic flow and deepens the spiritual dimension of the Tantric journey.

3. Sacred Sound Healing:

Integrate sacred sound healing into your Tantric massage practice. Utilize singing bowls, chimes, or vocal toning to create harmonious vibrations that resonate with the body's energy centers. Sound healing enhances the overall sensory experience, fostering a profound connection between the physical and spiritual realms.

4. Conscious Energy Exchange:

Elevate your Tantric practice by engaging in conscious energy exchange. As giver and receiver, visualize and intentionally exchange energetic currents during the massage. This practice deepens the sense of oneness and invites a heightened awareness of the subtle energies flowing between partners.

5. Sacred Geometry Visualization:

Incorporate sacred geometry visualization during the massage. Envision geometric patterns such as the Flower of Life or Sri Yantra in your mind's eye. As the giver, project these sacred symbols onto the receiver's body, fostering a meditative and energetically rich experience.

6. Shiva-Shakti Union:

Embrace the divine dance of Shiva and Shakti, embodying the union of masculine and feminine energies. Allow the roles of giver and receiver to fluidly interchange, transcending traditional gender dynamics. This practice invites a profound balance of energies, deepening the Tantric connection.

7. Extended Tantric Breathwork:

Expand your Tantric breathwork to include more intricate techniques. Experiment with circular breathing, breath retention, and synchronized breath cycles between giver and receiver. Advanced breathwork enhances energetic flow, heightens sensations, and fosters an even more intimate connection.

8.   Quantum Touch Healing:

Integrate Quantum Touch Healing principles into your Tantric massage practice. Focus on directing life force energy through your hands, facilitating physical and energetic healing. This advanced technique adds a therapeutic element to the massage, promoting balance and well-being.

9.   Sacred Union Meditation:

Conclude your Tantric massage sessions with a Sacred Union Meditation. As giver and receiver, sit in a shared meditation, visualizing a merging of energies and a deepening connection. This meditation amplifies the transformative power of the Tantric experience, transcending the physical realm.

10.   Cosmic Connection Integration:

Extend the Tantric experience beyond earthly dimensions with a Cosmic Connection Integration. Visualize your energies expanding beyond the confines of your physical bodies, merging with the cosmic energy of the universe. This advanced practice invites a transcendent and expansive connection between partners.

As you venture into these advanced Tantric practices, approach them with reverence, intention, and an open heart. Each technique serves as a gateway to deeper levels of connection, consciousness, and spiritual awakening. May your journey through these advanced practices be a sacred exploration, enriching the tapestry of your Tantric experience with profound intimacy and transformation.

7.1 Tantric Rituals

In the sacred tapestry of Tantric massage, rituals are the threads that weave intention, mindfulness, and spiritual connection into the fabric of the experience. These Tantric rituals imbued with ancient wisdom, invite practitioners to embark on a journey that transcends the physical and taps into the profound realms of the spiritual. Explore these Tantric rituals to deepen your connection with your partner and elevate the transformative power of your shared experience.

1.   **Temple Space Creation:**

Begin your Tantric ritual by creating a sacred temple space. Cleanse the environment, dim the lights, and adorn the space with symbolic elements such as candles, flowers, and sacred objects. This ritual establishes a consecrated atmosphere, inviting a sense of reverence and divine presence.

2.   Synchronized Breathwork Invocation:

Initiate the Tantric ritual with synchronized breathwork. Giver and receiver synchronize their breaths, creating a harmonious exchange of life force energy. This intentional breathwork serves as an invocation, inviting a sacred connection and aligning the energies of both partners.

3.   Anointing Ceremony with Sacred Oils:

Engage in an anointing ceremony using sacred oils. As the giver anoints the receiver, infuse the practice with reverence and intention. Choose oils with aromatic properties that enhance the sensory experience, fostering a deep connection with the spiritual and sensual aspects of the Tantric journey.

4.   Invocation of Divine Energies:

Incorporate an invocation of divine energies at the commencement of the Tantric massage. Giver and receiver can silently or verbally call upon the divine, setting the intention to invite sacred energies into the space. This ritual establishes a connection with higher realms, infusing the massage with spiritual significance.

5.   Chakra Activation and Balancing:

Prioritize chakra activation and balancing as a central Tantric ritual. Use intentional touch, energy awareness, and visualizations to activate and harmonize the seven energy centers within the body. This practice enhances the flow of spiritual energy, fostering a holistic and transformative experience.

6. Yab-Yum Meditation:

Incorporate the Yab-Yum meditation as a Tantric ritual. Giver and receiver sit in a position of intimate embrace, creating a union of masculine (Shiva) and feminine (Shakti) energies. This meditation deepens the connection, aligns polarities, and invites a transcendent experience of oneness.

7. Sacred Sound Resonance:

Integrate sacred sound resonance into your Tantric ritual. Use chanting, singing bowls, or mantras to create vibrational frequencies that resonate with the body's energy centers. The power of sound enhances the spiritual dimension of the massage, fostering a deeper connection with the divine.

8. Mudra Embodiment:

Embody Tantric mudras as a ritualistic aspect of the practice. The giver and receiver can adopt specific hand gestures that symbolize aspects of divine connection, unity, or spiritual principles. Mudras serve as a tangible expression of intention, enhancing the ritualistic nature of the Tantric experience.

9.   Intuitive Movement Exploration:

Engage in intuitive movement exploration as a ritual within Tantric massage. Allow the body to move organically, guided by the flow of energy and intuition. This spontaneous dance ritualizes the connection between the giver and the receiver, creating a fluid and dynamic exchange of energy.

10.   Transcendental Closing Blessing:

Conclude the Tantric ritual with a transcendental closing blessing. The giver and receiver can share words of gratitude, blessings, or affirmations. This closing ritual acknowledges the sacredness of the shared experience and invites the transformative energy to integrate into the spiritual essence of both partners.

As you infuse these Tantric rituals into your practice, embrace them with intention, presence, and an open heart. May each ritual become a gateway to the divine, deepening the spiritual connection and enriching the Tantric massage experience with profound significance.

7.2 Incorporating Meditation

Meditation, the art of cultivating presence and mindfulness, becomes a sacred companion in the Tantric massage journey. By seamlessly weaving meditation into the fabric of your practice, you invite a deeper connection with the self, the partner, and the transcendent energies that shape the Tantric experience. Explore these meditation practices to elevate your Tantric massage to new dimensions of consciousness and spiritual awakening.

1.   Mindful Breathing Meditation:

Commence your Tantric massage with a mindful breathing meditation. The giver and receiver sit together, focusing on the breath. Inhale and exhale intentionally, allowing the breath to become a unifying force. This meditation establishes a shared rhythm, fostering a sense of presence and connection.

2.   Loving-Kindness Meditation:

Integrate a Loving-Kindness Meditation into the Tantric experience. As the giver, silently offer thoughts of love, compassion, and well-being to the receiver. This meditation cultivates an atmosphere of warmth and acceptance, deepening the emotional and spiritual connection between partners.

3.   Body Scan Meditation:

Incorporate a Body Scan Meditation to enhance awareness and presence. The giver gently guides attention to each part of the receiver's body, fostering a deepening awareness of sensations. This meditation grounds the experience in the present moment, creating a profound connection between touch and consciousness.

4.   Visualization of Sacred Energy:

Engage in a Visualization Meditation that invokes sacred energy. Giver and receiver close their eyes, collectively visualizing a flow of divine energy entering and circulating through their bodies. This meditation amplifies the energetic exchange, connecting the Tantric experience to higher spiritual realms.

5.   Transcendental Breathwork Meditation:

Explore Transcendental Breathwork Meditation as a dynamic practice. Giver and receiver synchronize their breaths, gradually intensifying the rhythm. This meditation serves as a bridge to altered states of consciousness, deepening the spiritual dimension of the Tantric massage.

6.   Third Eye Activation Meditation:

Activate the third eye through meditation during the Tantric practice. As the giver, direct focused attention to the receiver's forehead, visualizing an opening of the third eye. This meditation heightens intuition and spiritual perception, fostering a connection with the higher realms.

7.   Unity Consciousness Meditation:

Invoke a sense of Unity Consciousness through meditation. Giver and receiver synchronize their breaths and visualize a merging of energies, transcending individual identities. This meditation facilitates a profound sense of oneness, elevating the Tantric experience to a shared spiritual journey.

8.   Intuitive Movement Meditation:

Integrate Intuitive Movement Meditation into your Tantric practice. Allow spontaneous, guided movement to arise naturally. The giver and receiver move with intention, expressing their connection through embodied meditation. This practice deepens the integration of mind, body, and spirit.

9.   Heart-Centered Meditation:

Center the Tantric experience on a Heart-Centered Meditation. Giver and receiver place their hands on each other's hearts, focusing on love and compassion. This meditation creates a heart-to-heart connection, infusing the massage with a profound sense of emotional and spiritual intimacy.

10. Sound Healing Meditation:

Conclude your Tantric massage with a Sound Healing Meditation. The giver and receiver engage in a meditative experience with soothing sounds, whether through instruments, chanting, or recorded vibrations. This meditation serves as a harmonious conclusion, grounding the shared spiritual journey.

As you embrace these meditation practices within your Tantric massage, may each moment of mindfulness become a gateway to higher states of consciousness and a deeper connection with the sacred essence of the Tantric experience. Through the union of meditation and touch, may you and your partner embark on a transformative journey of spiritual awakening and profound intimacy.

Chapter 8: Embarking on the Journey Together

As you and your partner venture into the sacred realms of Tantric massage, the journey becomes a shared odyssey of connection, exploration, and spiritual awakening. This chapter is a guide for partners seeking to deepen their bond through Tantric practices, fostering a harmonious union of mind, body, and spirit. Together, you will navigate the intricacies of intimacy, create sacred spaces, and embark on a transformative journey that transcends the ordinary and leads to profound connection.

1.   Mutual Intentions and Agreements:

Initiate your Tantric journey by establishing mutual intentions and agreements. Engage in open communication about your desires, boundaries, and expectations. By aligning your intentions, you create a foundation of trust and understanding, laying the groundwork for a harmonious Tantric experience.

2.   Co-Creating Sacred Spaces:

Embrace the art of co-creating sacred spaces. Together, infuse your environment with elements that evoke tranquility, such as candles, soft lighting, and soothing scents. This shared endeavor fosters a conducive atmosphere for Tantric exploration and deepens the sense of sacred connection.

3.   Partner-Bonding Rituals:

Incorporate partner-bonding rituals into your Tantric practice. Engage in activities that strengthen your connection, such as shared meditation, heartfelt conversations, or mutual acts of kindness. These rituals weave a tapestry of emotional intimacy, enhancing the depth of your connection beyond the boundaries of the Tantric massage.

4. Embracing Vulnerability Together:

Cultivate a space where vulnerability is not only accepted but embraced. Share your fears, desires, and insecurities. By creating a haven for vulnerability, you deepen your emotional connection, allowing the transformative power of Tantric massage to unfold with authenticity.

5. Exploring New Horizons:

Approach Tantric practices as an opportunity for joint exploration. Be open to trying new techniques, rituals, and meditations together. This shared curiosity fosters a sense of adventure, creating a dynamic and evolving Tantric journey that continuously deepens your connection.

6. Mindful Touch in Everyday Life:

Extend the practice of mindful touch into your everyday life. Incorporate intentional touches, hugs, and caresses outside of your Tantric sessions. This mindful touch becomes a continuous thread that weaves the energy of intimacy into the fabric of your relationship, fostering a lasting connection.

7.   Shared Breathwork Practices:

Explore shared breathwork practices as a means of enhancing your energetic connection. Engage in synchronized breathing, mirroring each other's breath, and experimenting with different breathwork techniques. These practices harmonize your energies, creating a profound sense of unity.

8.   Reflective Conversations:

Integrate reflective conversations into your Tantric journey. After each session, take time to share your experiences, insights, and emotions. These post-massage discussions deepen your understanding of each other and provide a platform for continued growth and connection.

9.   Cultivating Gratitude:

Make gratitude a cornerstone of your Tantric journey. Express appreciation for each other's presence, efforts, and vulnerability. Gratitude becomes a powerful force that amplifies the positive energy within your relationship, fostering a deep and reciprocal connection.

10. Setting Joint Intentions for Growth:

Conclude your Tantric journey sessions by setting joint intentions for growth. Discuss the aspects of your relationship that you both wish to nurture and enhance. These shared intentions become a roadmap for your continued journey, guiding you toward a more profound and enriched connection.

In embarking on the Tantric journey together, may your shared exploration be a celebration of love, intimacy, and spiritual awakening. As partners, may you weave a tapestry of connection that transcends the boundaries of the Tantric massage, creating a transformative and enduring journey that deepens your bond on every level.

8.1 Growing Together

As you navigate the intricate landscapes of Tantric massage with your partner, the journey becomes a dynamic process of growth and evolution. This section explores ways in which you and your partner can grow together, both individually and as a united force. Through mindful practices, shared experiences, and intentional efforts, the Tantric journey becomes a catalyst for personal development and the deepening of your connection.

1.   Cultivating Individual Awareness:

Encourage individual awareness as a foundation for growth. Both partners should embark on a journey of self-discovery, exploring personal desires, boundaries, and aspirations. Cultivating individual awareness lays the groundwork for a harmonious and enriching Tantric experience.

2.   Joint Meditation Practices:

Deepen your connection by engaging in joint meditation practices. Whether it's sitting together in silence, practicing mindfulness, or exploring guided meditations, shared moments of contemplation enhance your spiritual bond. Joint meditation becomes a vehicle for mutual growth and understanding.

3.   Embracing Change as a Couple:

Recognize that growth involves change, and embrace it as a couple. As you delve into Tantric practices, be open to evolving perspectives, desires, and boundaries. Embracing change together fosters resilience and adaptability, strengthening your connection amid the transformative journey.

4.   Mutual Support in Vulnerability:

Create a culture of mutual support in vulnerability. Acknowledge that personal growth often involves moments of discomfort and vulnerability. Be there for each other, providing a safe space to express fears, desires, and challenges. Mutual support becomes a catalyst for profound individual and collective transformation.

5. Setting Shared Goals:

Collaborate on setting shared goals within and outside the realm of Tantric massage. These goals can be personal, relational, or spiritual. Working towards common objectives creates a sense of unity and purpose, fostering a shared commitment to growth and development.

6. Reflective Journaling Together:

Engage in reflective journaling as a joint practice. After Tantric sessions or individual reflections, share your thoughts, insights, and aspirations. Reflective journaling becomes a shared narrative, documenting your journey and creating a space for mutual understanding and growth.

7. Integrating Tantric Principles in Daily Life:

Extend Tantric principles into your daily life. The mindfulness, presence, and connection cultivated during Tantric practices can permeate other aspects of your relationship. Applying Tantric principles in daily life becomes a continual source of growth and a reminder of the sacredness within your connection.

8. **Participating in Couples Workshops:**

Explore couples workshops and educational opportunities that align with Tantric philosophies. These experiences provide structured guidance and practices, offering new perspectives and tools for personal and relational growth. Couples workshops become shared spaces for learning and evolving together.

9. **Celebrating Milestones and Achievements:**

Celebrate milestones and achievements, both individual and shared. Acknowledge and honor the growth you've experienced together. Celebrations create positive reinforcement, fostering a sense of accomplishment and motivation for continued growth within your Tantric journey.

10. **Regular Relationship Check-Ins:**

Incorporate regular relationship check-ins into your routine. Use these check-ins to discuss your Tantric journey, individual growth, and the evolving dynamics within your relationship. Regular communication becomes a cornerstone for understanding, connection, and ongoing growth.

Through a commitment to individual awareness, shared practices, and intentional efforts, growing together within the Tantric journey becomes a transformative and enriching experience. May your shared path be one of continual evolution, deepening connection, and mutual support as you navigate the profound landscapes of personal and relational growth.

8.2 Integrating Tantric Principles into Daily Life

The essence of Tantric massage extends far beyond the confines of the massage room, reaching into the tapestry of your daily life. Integrating Tantric principles into your routine can foster a continuous connection, mindfulness, and a profound sense of sacredness. This section explores practical ways to infuse Tantric wisdom into your everyday existence, creating a harmonious and transformative lifestyle.

1.   **Mindful Morning Rituals:**

Begin your day with mindful morning rituals. Whether it's shared meditation, gentle stretches, or expressing gratitude, these rituals set a positive and intentional tone for the day ahead. Mindful mornings create a foundation for presence and connection that can extend throughout your daily activities.

2.   **Sacred Spaces at Home:**

Create sacred spaces within your home environment. Designate areas for meditation, reflection, or shared moments of connection. Adorn these spaces with elements that inspire tranquility, such as candles, cushions, and symbols that hold spiritual significance. Sacred spaces serve as constant reminders of the sacredness within your relationship.

3.   Conscious Mealtime Connection:

Transform mealtime into a conscious and connected experience. Share meals mindfully, savoring each bite and engaging in meaningful conversation. Use this time to express gratitude for the nourishment provided and the shared moments of connection, cultivating a deeper appreciation for the act of eating together.

4.   Mindful Touch and Affection:

Infuse mindful touch into your daily interactions. Incorporate gentle touches, hugs, or hand-holding throughout the day. These moments of affection become a continuous thread, reinforcing the energetic connection cultivated during Tantric massage. Mindful touch serves as a reminder of the sacredness within your physical connection.

5.   Shared Mindfulness Practices:

Engage in shared mindfulness practices. Whether it's a brief meditation, conscious breathing exercises, or moments of quiet reflection, practicing mindfulness together strengthens your connection and creates a sense of shared presence. These practices serve as touchpoints for grounding and reconnecting throughout the day.

6.   Tantric Communication:

Embrace Tantric principles in your communication. Prioritize active listening, speak from the heart, and express yourself authentically. Engage in heart-centered conversations that foster understanding and connection. Tantric communication becomes a transformative tool for deepening intimacy in everyday interactions.

7.   Energetic Awareness in Work and Play:

Maintain energetic awareness in your work and recreational activities. Whether you're engaged in professional pursuits or leisure, carry the principles of energetic connection and mindfulness with you. Being consciously present in various aspects of life allows Tantric wisdom to permeate every experience.

8.   Evening Connection Rituals:

Conclude your day with evening connection rituals. Share reflections on the day, express gratitude or engage in a brief meditation together. These rituals create a sense of closure, allowing you to transition from the activities of the day into a space of shared connection and intimacy.

9.   Sensory Exploration in Nature:

Connect with nature through sensory exploration. Take walks together, feel the earth beneath your feet, listen to the rustling of leaves, and appreciate the beauty around you. Nature becomes a canvas for heightened sensory experiences, allowing you to tap into the divine energy present in the natural world.

10. Intentional Bedtime Practices:

Infuse intention into your bedtime practices. Whether it's a brief gratitude ritual, a shared meditation, or simply expressing love and affection, intentional bedtime practices create a sacred space for connection before entering the realm of dreams. This conscious transition fosters a sense of unity as you embark on the journey of sleep together.

By integrating Tantric principles into your daily life, you transform routine activities into opportunities for connection, mindfulness, and spiritual growth. May your daily practices become a sacred dance that continuously deepens your bond, fostering a sense of harmony, presence, and shared spirituality in every moment.

Conclusion:

As we bring the journey of "Tantric Massage for Beginners: Awaken Your Senses, Deepen Intimacy, and Discover the Art of Sensual Connection" to a close, we find ourselves standing at the threshold of profound transformation. This exploration into the sacred realms of Tantric massage has been a voyage of self-discovery, connection, and awakening.

In these pages, we've delved into the ancient wisdom that lies at the heart of Tantric practices, unraveling the secrets of mindful touch, sacred rituals, and the fusion of physical and spiritual energies. From the foundational principles to the intricacies of advanced techniques, each chapter has been a guide, inviting you and your partner to embark on a journey that transcends the ordinary and taps into the extraordinary.

Tantric massage, as we've discovered, is not merely a physical experience—it's a dance of energies, a celebration of intimacy, and a pathway to spiritual connection. It's a journey that begins with individual self-awareness and expands into a shared exploration of the depths of partnership. Through conscious touch, mindful communication, and the integration of Tantric principles into daily life, you've been on the cusp of a profound transformation.

As you move forward, remember that Tantric massage is a living art, a canvas upon which you and your partner continually paint and explore. It's an ongoing dialogue between souls, an expression of love, and an ever-evolving dance of connection. The practices you've embraced are not confined to the massage room; they are threads that weave through the fabric of your daily existence, enriching each moment with the sacred energy of Tantric wisdom.

May this journey be a catalyst for a deeper understanding of yourself, your partner, and the limitless potential that lies within the union of mind, body, and spirit? May the art of sensual connection continue to awaken your senses, fostering a love that transcends boundaries and transforms the ordinary into the extraordinary.

In the tapestry of your shared experiences, may the spirit of Tantric massage linger—a reminder of the sacred dance you've embraced together. As you move forward, may this artful exploration be a source of continual growth, connection, and profound intimacy.

The odyssey of Tantric massage is not a destination but an ongoing pilgrimage—a journey where each touch, each breath, and each shared moment becomes a step toward a more conscious, connected, and vibrant existence. Embrace the art, savor the journey, and may the echoes of Tantric wisdom guide you on a lifelong exploration of sensual connection and spiritual awakening.

With love, awareness, and the eternal dance of energies,